AF207970

ASPARAGUS
CAN DO IT FOR YOU!

by
THEODORE A. BAROODY
*Ph.D. Nutrition, N.D., D.C.,
C.N.C.*

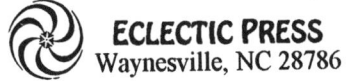

ECLECTIC PRESS
Waynesville, NC 28786

Look for other books available from
ECLECTIC PRESS
and Dr. Theodore A. Baroody

In natural food stores throughout the U.S.

Rose Baroody, editor
Nancy Baumgarten, copy editor
Lee Carper, cover illustration

*This reference work is based on research by the author. The opinions
expressed are purely opinions. It is not provided in order to diagnose,
prescribe or treat any disease, illness or injured condition of the body.
The author, publisher, printer, and distributors accept no
responsibility for such use. Any suggestions stated in this book are
in no way to be considered as a substitute for consultation with a
duly licensed doctor.*

ECLECTIC PRESS
205 Pigeon St.
Waynesville, NC 28786

TABLE OF CONTENTS

ASPARAGUS – MIRACLE OR PLAIN TRUTH?

Some things are just too good to be true. Then again, the simpler a truth is, the more it holds fast under intense scrutiny. The vegetable asparagus is one of these simple truths. Ingesting it in either food or food supplement form is both simple and produces remarkable health results. Yet, even though the use of asparagus may seem simple, the reasons for its wide range of health benefits are not.

In this book, we shall review the simple truth about all that asparagus can do. We shall also explore the complexities of why asparagus works from a research standpoint. Lastly, I shall share what I have seen in my practice from a clinical viewpoint.

We should all be encouraged by this book. For not only is asparagus accessible, it is available, usable and recommendable in all forms, except raw. The FDA, AMA, and their allied drug manufacturers cannot stop you from consuming it even if the information in this book should ever prove to be even slightly threatening to their multi-billion dollar industries.

In fact, asparagus is such a hardy and resilient plant that it grows wild in many countries, including the United States. Mrs. M. Grieve states that the southern steppes of Russia are covered with it as well as the southwest coast of England (1971).

I have heard that in some areas of the U.S.A. it is actually considered a nuisance that the "unenlightened" try to control with weed killers. Too bad they don't just cut, steam and eat it instead. The money they could save on medical bills and drugs would outweigh what they spent on weed killers 1000 to 1.

I am not saying that asparagus "cures" anything. Nor am I diagnosing. I leave curing and diagnosing to those who use drugs, surgery, and radiation. I offer you this statement from a wise man, "When the experts disagree, the rest of us are free to choose for ourselves." How often have you heard experts actually agree on anything? Yet you may end up agreeing with me about just how helpful asparagus can be.

HOW I FOUND OUT ABOUT THE BENEFITS OF ASPARAGUS

In 1971 I started traveling and studying extensively around the world. Healing in all forms was the thing I most studied. I eventually became a chiropractic student and simultaneously studied naturopathy. In 1979, I became acquainted with the work of a biochemist, Dr. Carey Reams (Gardner, 1979). He mentioned the use of asparagus to help regulate skipped heart beats (arrhythmias). Later, after graduating and wishing to help my own patients in any way I could, I recommended they eat asparagus for this common malady. It has worked in 95% of these cases over a 15 year period.

Over these same years, to my surprise, I began to notice many different types of symptoms relieved by asparagus as well. I then found a book by Dr. Richard

Broeringmeyer D.C., who spoke about a dentist, Dr. Vensel, who had cured himself of Hodgen's Disease (cancer) by eating asparagus daily. He also reported that a group of 60 cancer patients recovered their health by taking asparagus. Even in cases of benign tumors, asparagus has been found helpful. Dr. Broeringmeyer reported about a woman with a large internal tumor who began taking asparagus and within four weeks the tumor had reduced considerably. Then the lady contracted an intestinal virus and could not eat any asparagus for about five weeks. The tumor grew rapidly again. She then started taking the asparagus again until her doctor found her completely free of all symptoms. The tumor was gone. From this article and from my past experience with asparagus, I began to research all that I could find.

WHAT ASPARAGUS HELPS

The first recorded use of asparagus is found in ancient Ayurvedic medicine texts. This system has been practiced for 6000 years. In this most wondrous healing tradition, asparagus is highly regarded as the main Ayurvedic female reproductive tonic. It is listed as being highly nourishing, soothing, and calming to the heart. (Frawley, 1989)

Since Grecian times, the virtues of asparagus have been known as a diuretic, laxative and as a help for those who suffer from "symptoms of gravel and dropsy." It is mentioned by Cato the Elder in 200 B.C. and again by Pliny. It gained notice by the famous English herbalists Gerard and Culpepper in the 16th century. Then it was stated that when used as a decoction it "is good to clear the sight, and being held in the mouth easeth the toothache." Culpepper also tells us that it helps "those sinews that are shrunk by cramps and convulsions, and helpeth the sciatica." (Grieve, 1971)

Experiments done in 1739 indicated that asparagus would dissolve kidney stones and benefit all types of kidney disorders. (Gaumont, 1980) In 1854, a book called, **The Elements of Materia Medica** also stated that it was used as a popular remedy for kidney stones. (Adams, 1977)

It is most important to understand that I am making no health claims. Asparagus simply assists the body's energetic balance. So, from an energetic standpoint, I am stating the following things that it is presently reported by current practitioners to affect:

1) Reduces all kinds of tumors
2) Rebalances cardiac arrhythmias
3) Rebalances other heart imbalances
4) Removes chemical poisons
5) Removes heavy metal poisons
6) Clears the gall bladder ducts
7) Clears the pancreatic ducts
8) Clears the ureters
9) Removes kidney gravel that causes lower back pain all across the kidney areas, particularly in the early morning
10) Acts as a mild yet effective diuretic, reducing excessive swelling

11) Regulates the energetic rhythmic patterns that must exist between the heart and the kidney, thereby reducing pressure from the heart
12) Strengthens the overall kidney
13) Dissolves kidney stones (over a period of time)
14) Strengthens the liver
15) Dissolves gall bladder stones (over a period of time)
16) Reduces the feeling of heaviness in the brain

Swinburne Clymer, M.D., in **Diet, Key to Health** (1966), states that asparagus may support the body balance in situations such as:

1) Neurasthenia
2) Tuberculosis
3) Pus infections
4) Liver affections
5) Constipation
6) Tumors
7) Lack of recuperative power
8) Insomnia
9) Brain fatigue
10) Lifeless skin
11) Falling hair
12) Numbness

13) Depleted sexual system
14) Eye weakness
15) Tooth decay
16) Fatigue without cause
17) Abscesses
18) Neurotic tendencies
19) Mental confusion
20) Uneven pulse
21) Nerve exhaustion
22) Enlargement of the liver
23) Catarrh of bladder
24) Diabetes
25) Nervous excitement
26) Excessive flow during menopause

Gary Null (1973) a researcher, states that asparagus is also helpful for:
1) Stimulating the kidneys in a diuretic action
2) Mild laxative
3) Enlarged heart
4) Sedative for the nervous system
5) Conditions involving accumulation of fluids in tissues and body cavities

Food researcher and author, Anne-Marie Colbin (1986) states that asparagus is among the foods rich in folic acid, (vitamin B9). Folic acid triggers histamine production.

Correct histamine levels in either blood or tissues, are linked with the ability to achieve orgasm in both men and women. According to one source this would suggest that asparagus is a mild aphrodisiac. Recent studies that included 15,000 physicians as reported by Jane Brady in the *New York Times* and *Reader's Digest* suggest that folic acid appears critical in preventing some birth defects as well as helping ward off heart attacks, strokes and certain cancers. This is particularly true for tumors called adenomas which are the forerunners of colon cancer. Ms. Brady mentioned other studies that pointed out that low folic acid levels may increase the risk of lung and cervical cancer. This same article listed asparagus as one of the best sources of folic acid. This is because food sources of folic acid are much more readily available to the body than processed sources. (1994)

N.W. Walker (1970) states that asparagus juice breaks up oxalic acid crystals in the kidneys and throughout the muscular system making it good for rheumatism.

Dr. Marsh Morrison, D.C. uses asparagus, among other things, for his anti-arthritis program. He strongly encourages the consumption of asparagus spears daily for at

13

least three months and then to continue on after it has neutralized and eliminated much of the strong damaging acids. He reports that the safe, natural ammonia content in asparagus is highly alkaline which helps neutralize the poisons of a highly arthritic condition. (1982)

Dr. Broeringmeyer stated that asparagus will dissolve artery deposits (arteriosclerosis) and is a very effective parasite killer (vermifuge). At least two sources (Gaumont and Broeringmeyer) believe that certain DNA factors in asparagus help to make it effective in reaching into the cells.

I.E. Gaumont, a therapeutic researcher, states that asparagus contains histones which are believed to be active in controlling cell growth. He feels that asparagus has a substance that is a **cell growth normalizer**. This, he says, could account for its action on all types of cancer as well as acting as a overall body rejuvenator. (1980)

Organic plant information on histones indicate that its DNA factors are similar to human strains.

In Holland, Dr. Cornelius Moerman, M.D. devised a *nutritional approach for cancer that won government approval.* He concluded that there were eight substances vital to ideal health:

1) Vitamin A
2) Vitamin C
3) B-Complex
4) Vitamin E
5) Citric Acid
6) Iodine
7) Iron
8) Sulphur

By using these as he suggested and following his dietary program, many hundreds of hopeless cases have been helped. (Jochems, 1990)

An incredible coincidence occurred to me as I researched the constituents of asparagus and the above diet. Seven of the eight substances Dr. Moerman mentioned were all present in asparagus. Only vitamin E was missing. However, in my practice when a vitamin E need shows in a client and they take asparagus, no other vitamin E supplement is needed to correct the deficiency. So I suspect that pure organic asparagus makes the vitamin E pathway available so that vitamin E can be absorbed into the body. I cannot definitively state that all the conditions listed in this chapter will be helped. However, asparagus obviously has worked for many people in the past with all kinds of problems. Sally Koslow, editor-in chief of *McCall's Magazine* writes, "Add asparagus to your menu. Stock up on this cancer-fighting vegetable. . ." (April 1995). Since mainstream America is now becoming aware of asparagus, why not take it daily and see what it does for you?

VITAMINS & MINERALS IN ASPARAGUS

The vitamins, minerals and other substances found in asparagus that I have been able to identify from previously noted research are:

1) Arsenic (organic chelated)
2) Calcium
3) Potassium
4) Sodium
5) Magnesium
6) Iron
7) Phosphorus
8) Chlorine
9) Sulphur
10) Silicon
11) Iodine
12) Bromine
13) Zinc
14) Vitamin A
15) Thiamine (B1)
16) Riboflavin (B2)
17) Niacin (B3)

18) Folic Acid (B9)
19) Vitamin C
20) Citric Acid
21) L-Asparagine
22) Asparagusic acid (Gives part of the ammonia smell in urine. It breaks down into a highly alkaline forming ammonia-like compound.)

One source (Gaumont, 1980) actually lists all of the B-complex family as a component. Even though it has not been confirmed through standard analysis methods, a thorough clinical test with applied kinesiology, has been able to show that when serious client imbalances displayed the need for the entire B-complex, and asparagus was given, that not only did it quickly correct the kinesiological imbalance, but stabilized all related B-complex deficiency symptoms as well.

I am sure the above list is incomplete, since I have observed too many difficult clinical situations that asparagus has rebalanced beyond what these substances are known to correct. At this time, however, every substance that has been found by credible sources to **actually be in** asparagus, I have reported.

THE GOOD IN ARSENIC

There is one greatly misunderstood **organically chelated** element that the body possesses in small amounts and **must** have to live. That element is arsenic. Let me make it clear that I am not speaking about arsenic in its inorganic life-threatening form.

The properties of bioavailable arsenic already present in the body are as follows:

1) **It is released during the presence of tumors.**

2) It is mostly concentrated in the liver where it is released as needed into the bloodstream.

3) It is released during menstruation and during the fifth and sixth months of pregnancy.

4) It is a constituent of living cells found also in the epidermis, hair, nails, thyroid glands, breasts and brain (in conjunction with iodine)

5)   It has a chemical affinity for phosphorous and harmonizes with iodine. (Jensen, 1983)

Dr. Reams found organic arsenic in its most bioavailable and assimilable form in our now familiar friend, asparagus. He stated that the bioavailable traces of arsenic will stabilize a skipping heart. **He also said that organic dietary arsenic is as important and necessary to the heart as iron is to the liver.** Although this may sound too incredible to believe, there may be some truth to it. Simple truth.

I have watched this treatment help scores of people with cardiac arrhythmia with no danger and no side effects. A good number of these people had been told that it was hereditary, or that they just had to live with it even when medications didn't work.

Several cardiologists, I consulted, reported that conservative figures for cardiac arrhythmia in our population were 70% for those over 65 years of age and 30% for those below 65. This translates into one person in three under 65 and 2 out of 3 that are over 65. And remember these are conservative figures. This includes testing either by simple blood pressure and pulse tests or by more sophisticated procedures such as electrocardiogram. Further, the medical community does not feel every type of arrhythmia to be a problem. Since many of these arrhythmias are transient they don't consider them to be dangerous. In my own work, I feel that **any** arrhythmia is an indicator of energetic-body imbalance. It is a symptom of deeper problems and if at all possible should be corrected.

Through his extraordinary scientific research, Dr. Phillip Callahan, an entomologist and interdisciplinary researcher (1984), has shown that the human heart has a particular radio wave frequency. As long as this frequency is maintained, every cell in the body stays in balance. Once out of rhythm, the frequency is altered, thereby energetically altering every organ, gland and cell in the body. Eventually, this would lead to some dis-ease process that would become more noticeable to the afflicted person. (personal conversation, 1992)

I have tested Callahan's idea again and again and found that once heart balance is restored, health inevitably follows.

THE SPECIALNESS OF ASPARAGINE

Asparagus contains a special amino acid - Asparagine. **It was the first amino acid ever discovered.** This was accomplished in 1806 by Vauqelin and Robiquet who succeeded in separating it from asparagus juice. (Robinson, 1980)

Chemically, L-Asparagine looks like this: $H_2NOCCH_2CH(NH_2)CO_2H$. But don't let this imposing string of letters and numbers scare you. It really means something good. Through its action, asparagine can release positive energy into the body and then metabolize it into aspartic acid. This is important because aspartic acid assists two of the body's most important metabolic pathways.

The first pathway is the urea cycle which is the foundation of nitrogen metabolism. Aspartic acid (from asparagine)

23

is an active brain neurotransmitter in the cerebellum, hippocampus and hypothalamus. Asparagusic acid, a cyclic disulfate (2,2' - dithioisobutyric acid) is reported to be the main sulfur compound that gives asparagus its unique flavor and post-digestion urinary odor. You can "smell" it working when you urinate. This is normal. The odor is the result of the specialness of asparagus changing the body chemistry and eliminating wastes while it breaks down its constituents of nitrogen, sulphur, and ammonia. Aspartic acid can be prepared from asparagine by acid hydrolysis. (Robinson, 1980)

The second pathway that aspartic acid assists is carbohydrate metabolism. Cell metabolism is also enhanced by the utilization of aspartic acid. It is as though there were a special something in asparagus that has the ability to actually reach into the heart of a cell and positively affect its most basic genetic nature. (Feiser, 1961)

After reviewing the foregoing available material on asparagus, I am bewildered as to why present day researchers and doctors have not explored all the potential health benefits of asparagus.

ASPARAGUS AS AN ANTIOXIDANT

As a natural result of your body's use of oxygen, a waste factor is created called free radicals. Free radicals are extremely unstable tiny molecular fragments. They combine with unsaturated fats to form peroxides which damage cells and cell walls. They are your body's death squad. The destruction free radicals create is cumulative over the years, causing everything from age spots and wrinkling to terminal illnesses. When healthy, the body will eliminate most excess free radicals. Yet, with the stresses and poor foods of this day and time **our natural protectors, antioxidants**, are overused and under supplied by the body.

Antioxidants are substances that knock out free radicals, thus affording cellular protection. Asparagus, particularly in its pure organic form, contains the several elements necessary to eliminate free radicals. The most important of these is the alkaloid asparagine. It is becoming recognized as a very effective highly assimilable, and bioavailable antioxidant when taken in its natural organic form. (Wade, 1987)

Vitamins A and C, also found in asparagus, are the other antioxidants that work synergistically in a perfect balance with the body. According to Carlson Wade the minerals of iron and sulphur, (also found in asparagus) create antioxidant action by cleansing away fatty deposits and free radicals from your gastrointestinal area and help to cast out wastes from infected cells. A portion of what you smell in your urine is the free radicals being eliminated. To my knowledge, there is no other completely natural, whole food that causes this obvious urinary odor which is indicative of tissue acid waste and free radical elimination.

I have never found a safer, more effective, nor less expensive antioxidant than asparagus. It works steadily and mildly bringing protection from the free radicals that can destroy cellular tissues and set the stage for disease in the body.

THE ALKALINE-FORMING POWER OF ASPARAGUS

In my book **Alkalize Or Die**, I go into detail about the importance of maintaining the body's alkaline/acid ratios. The huge health problems of our times are largely the result of our highly acid-forming diets. The countless names attached to the illnesses do not really matter. What does matter is that they all come from the same root cause . . . . **too much tissue acid waste in the body!**

Waste acids that are not eliminated when they should be are reabsorbed from the colon into the liver and put back into general circulation. They then deposit in the tissues. **It is these tissue acid residues that create pain and sickness of all kinds!** Tissue acid poisons are the prime food sources for bacteria, fungus, and parasites, which cause tremendous problems as they are allowed to get out of balance. All this equates to great overall illness.

Pure organic asparagus is a very highly alkaline-forming substance. Its ability to quickly change the PH of the body is evidenced by how rapidly you can smell it in your urine after you eat it.

In every source I can find, asparagus is considered in the top number of most alkaline-forming foods. This fact along with all its other health-giving attributes makes the daily use of pure organic asparagus a very sensible idea.

Let pure asparagus help you in your quest for a better long-term alkaline forming lifestyle. Acidify yourself and suffer; alkalize yourself and stay well.

HOW TO USE IT

The first thing to remember is: DO NOT EAT RAW, UNCOOKED ASPARAGUS. Asparagus is very potent in raw form, containing an active enzyme that if eaten in any sizeable amount can cause problems. (Gaumont, 1980)
You have two options:

1) You can buy frozen, canned or fresh asparagus. (*Green Giant or Stokeley* brands seem to be the purest). To prepare, blend either fresh steamed asparagus or store-bought canned or frozen asparagus and eat daily.

2) The other option is to use organically-grown Aspara-Can[R] capsules which contain no salt, sugar, wheat, soy, flavorings, or preservatives of any kind. Aspara-Can[R] is heated just enough to kill the active enzyme and still maintain all the other positive attributes.

DOSAGES: If symptoms are severe: Take 8 to 12 tablespoons of the asparagus puree daily, 4 to 6 tablespoons at breakfast and 4 to 6 at supper. *OR* take 8 to 12 Aspara-Can capsules daily. If symptoms are mild to moderate: Take 4 to 6 tablespoons of the asparagus puree daily *OR* take 4 to 6 Aspara-Can capsules.

As a preventive measure: Take 3 to 4 tablespoons of the asparagus puree *OR* take 3 to 4 Aspara-Can capsules daily. *(One tablespoon of asparagus puree equals one Aspara-Can capsule. There are approximately 13 to 15 tablespoons of puree in a can of asparagus.*

SIDE EFFECTS: None ever reported by others. I have noted on rare occasions that as the body is beginning to heal, the kidneys and low back will ache all the way across. This is very temporary and indicates that large amounts of kidney gravel and other tissue acid waste poisons are working through. Drink distilled water and add fresh lemon juice to help these flush through.

LENGTH OF TIME: 6 months to 1 year OR until your doctor finds all tests negative <u>and</u> you feel all symptoms gone.

RESPONSE TIME: Depending on severity, you will usually feel some improvement within 2 to 4 weeks. It is my recommendation to continue taking it while symptoms persist. And most importantly: DO NOT SKIP! TAKE IT EVERY DAY! After you feel better you may cut back to every other day. Most people will not be consistent with cooking and eating it every day for long periods of time, so I formulated Aspara-Can because it is easier to take. Who really knows whether what you get out of a can or jar is preservative free? With the allowances I have seen given to the food industry, I just do not trust them. Many are still allowed to add ingredients in spite of their claims. Salt is added to most canned foods which can be unbeneficial for high blood pressure.

There are very few days in my office when I do not hear a good report about what either eating or taking asparagus is doing for my clients and their friends. Daily I find that it is useful for some situation that I previously had no idea it would help.

I use Aspara-Can as an indicator for how well I am doing. Through muscle-testing, I can see if the dosage needed by my body has increased or decreased. If it has increased, I know I am accumulating too many dangerous acid wastes and free radicals. If it has stayed the same or decreased, I am under less overall systemic stress from these aging poisons.

Muscle-testing is an art, not a science. It takes practice to learn. You will be surprised, however, at how fast you can become good at it for yourself, spouse and friends. If you don't want to use muscle testing, just follow the guidelines given under "dosages."

Muscle-testing is done as follows:

1)   Say a prayer to clear your mind and heart. This will allow the test to be valid. Also, you must stay in this prayerful attitude while testing.

2)   Have the person you are testing extend their arm to the side.

3)   Put the amount of Aspara-Can to be tested in their other hand. For

example, start with four capsules (the recommended dosage).

4) Push down on their arm with a very light pressure. You will be able to feel their strength. If their arm drops, four is too many. Try three and retest. If three is tested and the arm is strong then that is the number the person needs for that day.

5) If their arm is strong at four go to five, then six or until the arm goes weak. When the arm is weak, say at ten, back down to nine and retest. If the arm is strong, then the person needs nine a day.

CLIENT AND PATIENT REPORTS

The following studies are only a tiny fraction of what I have seen asparagus do first hand.

Ms. K.H. had suffered from intense episodes of gall bladder and colon pain. She had been to every type of doctor, and in the hospital with no results. Though I had treated her and it helped temporarily, the pain would return. After I started using asparagus, I told her about it and had occasion to give her some right in the office while she was having an acute attack. The pain completely disappeared in under three minutes. Now she can control the pain while the asparagus continues working to clean out her various ducts.

Mr. G.S. suffered from lumbago. Adjustments had not helped. I tried colonics and a group of other food supplements. After starting on asparagus, he reports his "rheumatiz" is much improved.

Mr. T.H. who is in his eighties, was suffering from high blood pressure and frequent heart-skipping. None of his medications, though often changed, seemed to help. After three months on asparagus, his blood pressure was 126 over 77 and there was no heart-skip. Also, many of his frequent arthritic pain episodes disappeared.

Mrs. C.Z. was suffering from lower back pain around her kidneys and into her left hip. I found this to be kidney gravel. After taking asparagus, the pain diminished. Also a right breast tumor that she had completely *disappeared* during this time, though I was not treating her for cancer. I was only trying to rebalance the body.

Ms. M.W. presented me with all her blood work. She was diagnosed by her medical doctor with a severe kidney problem and a very low creatinine level. I recommended Aspara-Can. In one month the creatinine level returned completely to normal and her kidney problem disappeared.

She said her doctor was amazed and I told her I was too.

Mrs. M.C., a nurse, had been diagnosed with a large breast tumor by her medical doctor. I gave her Aspara-Can to help with her imbalanced heart beat. After two months, the heart normalized. The breast tumor, which I do not treat, reduced by over 60%. She is continuing to take this harmless vegetable to stabilize her heart.

Mrs. T.M. came to me with a serious leg infection, having considerable dark discoloration in one area and red, painful inflammation in another. Drugs of various types had only been helping a little, then would stop working. Knowing that asparagus contains asparagine, a very effective, yet "safe" antioxidant, and that some researchers have used it to clear out all kinds of infections, I recommended Aspara-Can. The results were dramatic. At two weeks, the red inflammation was mostly gone. At four weeks, the long-time dark discoloration started to break up. At six weeks, the inflammation was gone with only two small scabs left and the discoloration of old blood barely noticeable.

Mr. D.D. had been medically diagnosed with an enlarged prostate. He was in considerable discomfort upon sitting. After 1 month on asparagus his pain had subsided and his discomfort on sitting was greatly reduced.

Mrs. C.R. showed me her hands. They were scaly, cracked open and bleeding in many places. She told me she had tried drugs, lotions and all kinds of vitamin and minerals from several different doctors. All of this had not helped. I gave her the Aspara-Can and did not see her again for about 3 months. She returned and showed me her hands. The cracks and bleeding were gone, but the scaliness remained. Her story, however, confirmed the specialness of asparagus. She said that **all** the itching, scaling and cracked bleeding had disappeared. Then she ran out of Aspara-Can over the Christmas holidays and all the symptoms returned. Upon taking it again, the symptoms were once again leaving and the remaining scaliness was fast disappearing for a second time.

If pure organic asparagus is doing this for Mrs. C.R.'s very obvious symptoms, imagine all the good it is doing unseen for the rest of her body.

Mrs. Betty M. has severe allergy attacks. She came in the office during one of these attacks. She was having chest tightness, burning eyes, and painful muscle spasms in her neck. I gave her Aspara-Can and the pain disappeared in about 2 minutes along with all the other symptoms. Now she uses it daily and as needed when she gets into an exposure of some allergen. She states she "no longer feels like a helpless victim of her environment." Also, a long-term, persistent pain at the base of her thumb, medically diagnosed as arthritis, completely stopped in one hour after taking the Aspara-Can.

Mrs. S.S., 78 years old, came in to see me with a very irregular heart beat. It was fast then slow, then skipped and finally beat very hard. She felt as though she were having a heart attack. After two months on Aspara-Can, her heart was steady and regular. Her blood pressure was normal, and according to her medical doctor the heaviness and fluid retention around her heart had diminished to normal. He was amazed and pleased at her progress. She reported she felt like a 25 year old again.

Mrs. C.B. has very intense migraine headaches. I gave her Aspara-Can for her irregular heart. She reported that whenever she took it during a headache it would relieve the pain quicker and better than drugs.

Mrs. S.G., age 40 came to me with a medically diagnosed hiatal hernia and carpal tunnel syndrome. She also suffered from very excessive gas and a great deal of swelling, particularly noticeable in her hands. She had been to over 15 doctors and had tried every drug available and every over the counter substance known. She reacted violently to all of them. Mrs. S.G. is one of the many highly-sensitive individuals in the world who reacts to everything. I started her on food supplements and over a 2 year period tried numerous protocols while carefully documenting her case. Nothing worked. Just like before, she reacted negatively. Even though I have manipulated over 5,000 hiatal hernia syndrome victims in my work (see my book **Hiatal Hernia Syndrome**) I was not able to do more than give her temporary relief from this devastating malady. Out of desperation, more than anything else, I suggested Aspara-Can. I figured that it being a whole unprocessed food, perhaps her body would accept it. After two weeks, she came in beaming, "Look at my hands! All the swelling is gone. I can get my rings off again. Many of my friends have noticed how much better they are." The pain at the base of her thumb, diagnosed as carpal tunnel syndrome, had

40

also vanished. She further reported that her digestive pain from the hiatal hernia had stopped and that her excessive gas was gone.

Mr. J.Z. is not a patient. He had heard about the benefits of asparagus from someone else, bought it from us and took it for several weeks. He came in the office to report to me the disappearance of a large group of persistent skin cancers on his head. Usually he would go quite often to the dermatologist to get them burned off. This time, after taking Aspara-Can, and the cancers disappeared, he decided to stop taking it and they returned. Upon starting asparagus again, the cancers readily disappeared. His wife says his skin looks the best it has in 10 years. He also mentioned that the brown spots on his arm were disappearing.

Mr. R.L. is not a patient, but his story is fascinating. Over sixty years ago he was a young boy in serious condition with Rheumatic Fever. His doctors expected him to die any moment. There was nothing else to do for him. However, someone knew something about asparagus and fed him an almost exclusive diet of it three times a day with no other medication. After 6 months he was completely well. Obviously, someone knew the benefits of asparagus and this knowledge saved his life.

My personal experience with asparagus had been for preventive maintenance... or so I thought. My lower back would hurt in the early morning. I felt this was the result of a spinal accident I had had 15 years before. The discomfort would stop after arising and moving around. I used to have special bedding, and sleeping in hotel rooms or other people's homes was very uncomfortable. After three months of taking Aspara-Can capsules daily, I have been able to sleep much more comfortably on almost any bed. What I thought was a spinal problem was really a condition of kidney congestion and possibly a localized infection. Also, because of improved kidney function, overall morning stiffness and swelling has vanished.

My assistant, Mrs. P.C. was having the same problem with her back in the early morning. When she heard I was better, she started on Aspara-Can and her long-time early morning back pain (that she had been blaming on her bed) had disappeared too.

Three other enlightening cases reported by Rex Adams in his book, **Miracle Medicine Foods**, (1977) pages 25 and 65 are:

On March 5, 1971, a lung victim was put on the operating table where they found (disease) so widely spread that it was inoperable. The surgeons sewed him up and declared his case hopeless. On April 5, he heard about asparagus therapy and immediately started taking it. By August, x-ray pictures revealed that all signs of the tumors had disappeared.

One woman reported that asparagus therapy cured her kidney disease which started in 1949. She had over 30 operations for kidney stones and was receiving government disability payments for "a terminal kidney condition." She attributes the cure of this kidney trouble entirely to the asparagus therapy.

A 68 year old businessman had suffered from bladder trouble for sixteen years. After years of medical treatments, including cobalt radiation, without improvement, he went on asparagus. Within three months, hospital examinations revealed that his bladder tumor had disappeared and that his kidneys were normal.

Many people report to me that taking asparagus just "feels" right. They recognize it is doing something positive for their health even if they are not sure what it is.

I plan to consume asparagus for the rest of my life. I am convinced that it is helping many small problems of which I am not even aware, until one day I notice they have disappeared. It is a completely natural, whole, untampered-with food. Being powerful, yet non-toxic, it works with each individual according to the natural laws of the body. Because it is a pure food, the body knows exactly what to do and where it is most needed. Therefore asparagus assists the body in cleansing, correctly readjusting its many biochemical processes, and healing at the proper rate for each person. Every little nook and cranny of the body then gets a good alkaline scrubbing, which revives health by eliminating toxins.

CONCLUSION

In conclusion, I would like to state that the remarkable results I see with heart-skipping alone is reason enough to consider the benefits of eating or taking asparagus. Cardiac arrhythmia is a very widespread problem. Both benign and dangerous types exist. The exact figures for this are unknown. Senior citizens suffer the most, yet all ages are affected.

I am not recommending asparagus to you for any phase of cancer. It may however, offer some help in prevention of this problem. Never stop your drugs nor consider replacing them with asparagus without your doctor's knowledge and consent. Yet don't let your doctor or your common sense overlook something as simple and potentially healthful as taking asparagus.

From all the research I reviewed, it appears that no one knows for sure why asparagus works for so many different conditions. Is it the synergistic effects of its powerful antioxidant properties? Is it the arsenic which is also released by the liver when tumors arise? Is it asparagine that regulates and readjusts two of the most important pathways in the body, increasing oxygen in the cells which then seems to help life-threatening situations? Is it the unique combination of the thirteen known minerals and six known vitamins? Is it the very high alkaline-forming content of asparagus that counters the very acid conditions of arthritis and terminal illnesses? Or is it some type of holy blessing that we have been given by our Heavenly Father -- a simple truth, growing inauspiciously in our gardens and along our roadsides?

May good health and longevity be yours!

REFERENCES

Adams, Rex - **Miracle Medicine Foods**, West
Nyack, NY: Parker Publishing Co., 1977

Andersen, Arden B. - **Science in Agriculture**,
Kansas City, MO: Acres U.S.A., 1992

Baroody, Theodore A. - **Alkalize or Die**,
Waynesville, NC: Eclectic Press, 1990

Baroody, Theodore A. - **Hiatal Hernia Syndrome**,
Waynesville, NC: Eclectic Press, 1987

Brady, Jane E. - Reprinted article from **New York
Times** and **Reader's Digest** - "Folic Acid,
Superstar?" Pleasantville, NY: Reader's
Digest Association, June 1994

Braverman, Eric R. and Pfeiffer, Carl C. The **Healing Nutrients Within**, New Canaan, CT: Keats Publishing, 1987

Broeringmeyer, Richard - **The Problem Solver Nutritionally Speaking**, Murray, KY: Self-published, 1977

Callahan, Philip S. - **Ancient Mysteries, Modern Visions**, Kansas City, MO: Acres U.S.A., 1984

Clymer, R. Swinburne - **Diet - A Key to Health**, Philadelphia: Franklin Publishing, 1966

Colbin, Annemarie - **Food & Healing**, New York, NY: Ballantine Books, 1986

Fieser, Louis F. and Fieser, Mary - **Advanced Organic Chemistry**, New York, NY: Reinhold Publishing, 1961

Frawley, Dr. David, O.M.D. - **Ayurvedic Healing**, Salt Lake City, Utah: Passage Press, 1989

Gardner, Stanley & Gertrude - **Alphabetical Reference Manual**, Washington, IA: Self-published, 1979

Gaumont, I.E. - **Nine-Day Inner Cleansing and Blood Wash for Renewed Youthfulness and Health**, West Nyack, NY: Parker Publishing Co., 1980

Grieve, M. - **A Modern Herbal**, New York, NY: Dover Publications, Inc., 1971

Hawkins, Harold F. - **Applied Nutrition**, La Habra, CA: Mojave Books, 1947

Heritage, Ford - **Composition & Facts About Foods**, Mokelumne Hill, CA: Health Research, 1971

Jensen, Bernard - **The Chemistry of Man**, Escondido, CA: Self-published, 1983

Jensen, Bernard - **Food Healing for Man**, Escondido, CA: Self-published, 1983

Jochems, Ruth - **Dr. Moerman's Anti-Cancer Diet**, Garden City Park, NY: Avery Publishing Group, 1990

MacFadden, Bernarr - **The Encyclopedia of Health**, New York, NY: MacFadden Publishing Co., 1933

Manthei, Joseph C. - **More Excellent Way Ministries - Vols. 1, 2 and 3**, Drumore, PA: Self-published, 1981

Morrison, Marsh - **Doctor Morrison's Amazing Healing Foods: With Miracle Health Promoter M**, West Nyack, NY: Parker Publishing Co., 1982

49

Mowrey, Daniel B. - **The Scientific Validation of Herbal Medicine:** Cormorant Books, 1986

Null, Gary and Null, Steve - **The Complete Handbook of Nutrition,** New York, NY: Dell Publishing, 1973

Robinson, Trevor - **The Organic Constituents of Higher Plants,** North Amherst, MA: Cordus Press, 1980

Wade, Carlson - **Eat Away Illness,** West Nyack, NY: Parker Publishing Co., 1987

Walker, N.W. - **Raw Vegetable Juices,** Phoenix, AZ: Norwalk Press, 1970

PRODUCTS AND BOOKS BY DR. BAROODY

ALKALIZE OR DIE $14.95
This eye-opening book will help you discover what causes tissue wastes, how to prevent maladies using foods that create alkalinity. Includes 21 day menu planner, 55 recipes and alkaline/acid adjustment scale. 2nd printing. Health food stores rave about it. Hippocrates Institute uses it as a teaching tool.   ISBN: 0-9619595-3-3

HIATAL HERNIA SYNDROME: $ 9.95
Insidious Link to Major Illness
The only comprehensive self-help book on hiatal hernias. Documents 45 unsuspected symptoms contributing to many modern day ills. Pictures and diagrams make it easy to use. Popular book for over 8 years, 4th printing.
                    ISBN: 0-9619595-2-5

ASPARAGUS CAN DO IT FOR YOU! $ 4.95
Informative book on old and new research about the amazing health benefits of asparagus. Explains exactly how to use it and why it is important to everyone.
                    ISBN: 0-9619595-4-1

ASPARA-CAN^R CAPSULES $12.95
500 mg. of pure organic asparagus (asparagus officinalis) 100 Capsules

H.H.S. FORMULA^R $13.95
After working with thousands of Hiatal Hernia Syndrome sufferers worldwide, Dr. Baroody formulated this special product for total digestive system support. Contains 16 correctly balanced enzymes, herbs, vitamins, minerals and extracts. 100 Capsules

ORDER FORM

Name _____

Street _____

City _____ State _____ Zip _____

Send check or money order to:
HEALTHY ALTERNATIVES, LLC
205 Pigeon St., Waynesville, NC 28786
1-800-566-1522

Book Titles/Product	Qty	Each	Total
Alkalize or Die	____	$14.95	____
Hiatal Hernia Syndrome	____	~~9.95~~	____
Asparagus Can Do It For You	____	~~4.95~~	____
Aspara-Can^R Capsules	____	~~12.95~~	____
H.H.S. Formula^R	____	~~~~	____

SHIPPING AND HANDLING:
(All orders sent U.P.S.)

under $15	$3.50
$ 15.01 - 35.00	4.00
$ 35.01 - 55.00	4.50
$ 55.01 - 75.00	5.00
$ 75.01 - 95.00	5.50
$ 95.01 - 115.00	6.00
$115.01 - 135.00	6.50
Over $135.00	FREE

Call for shipping rates outside U.S.A.
Canadian shipments are double above

Subtotal: _____

Shipping
(See box): _____

NC residents add 6%
Sales tax: _____

TOTAL _____

Credit Card # _____ exp. date _____

Signature _____